The
Parke-Davis
Manual
on
EPILEPSY

Useful Tips That Help You Get the Best Out of Life

Consulting Medical Editors

Solomon L. Moshé, MD

Professor of Neurology
Neuroscience and Pediatrics
Albert Einstein College of Medicine
Montefiore Medical Center
Bronx, New York

John M. Pellock, MD

Professor of Neurology
and Pediatrics
Director of Epilepsy Clinics
Medical College of Virginia
Virginia Commonwealth University
Richmond, Virginia

Matthew C. Salon, MD

Section of Neurology
Munson Medical Center
Traverse City, Michigan

The Parke-Davis Manual on Epilepsy
A KSF Group Publication

PRINTING HISTORY
First U.S. edition published December 1992

ISBN 0-9634953-1-3
Library of Congress Catalog Card Number: 92-74838

PRINTED IN THE UNITED STATES OF AMERICA

Pharmaceutical products cited in the text are trademarks that are
registered by their respective companies.

Editorial Director, John Norwood.
Publisher, Aryeh Rubin.
Senior Editor, Greg Bezkorovainy. Senior Associate Editor, Monique Lui.
Associate Editor, Debra Averick. Assistant Editors, Pamela Cañate, Mark
Chesnut. Editorial Assistants, Wendy Klein, Elena Ratushewitz. Project
Director, Karen Hunt. Project Assistant, Mary Schrader. Assistant to the
Publisher, Cheryl Cohen. Communications Assistant, Kira O'Day. Con-
troller, Barbara Kelly. Director of Sales, John J. Racik. Artwork, Matthew
Archambault.

The purpose of this book is to provide useful, timely information to people
who have epilepsy. There is a dearth of such information written for
patients, and we hope this book will help fill that void. In so doing, we hope
to foster a more informed patient–physician bond and a greater apprecia-
tion of the importance of compliance with physicians' instructions.

This book is designed to inform the reader about matters relating to epilepsy
and to offer practical suggestions for an improved quality of life. The
publisher and sponsors of this book do not offer medical services. It is the
intention of the publication to augment the services of the physician and to
encourage its readers to obtain professional medical advice on any health-
related matters. The opinions and recommendations stated in this publication
are not necessarily endorsed by the editors, publisher, sponsors, or editorial
review board.

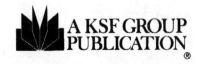

A KSF GROUP PUBLICATION
®

Parke-Davis Pharmaceuticals

People know a lot more about epilepsy now than ever before. And maybe the most important thing doctors and patients have learned is that there's a better chance of controlling seizures and thus living life to its fullest when the patients are well informed.

At Parke-Davis, we're sincerely committed to helping doctors and patients work together to keep epilepsy under control. For over 50 years, Parke-Davis has led the scientific community in epilepsy research, and we've put all those years of experience into this book.

Here's the information you need, the information you've asked for, to help you live life to its fullest. And the more you know and the greater your number of resources, the better your chances of successfully controlling and coping with epilepsy.

Everything in this book is designed to make it useful and easy to use. We've even included an Encyclodex, a special index that tells you what epilepsy-related words mean and where to find the words in the book.

As you read the manual, you'll have the peace of mind that the information you're getting is on the mark: The manual's editorial advisory board boasts some of the brightest minds in neurology.

Parke-Davis dedicates this book to you. With it, we hope to help you work with your doctor to control epilepsy and ensure that you have the opportunity to live life to its fullest.

CONTENTS

1 OVERVIEW

Many people don't realize how common epilepsy really is. This is partly due to the good control of epilepsy that people usually have. But the fact is that somewhere around 2 million Americans are affected by epilepsy.

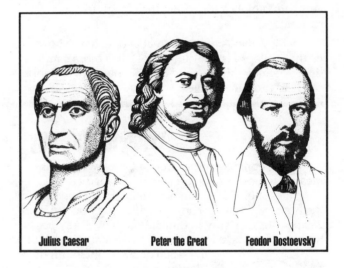

Julius Caesar   Peter the Great   Feodor Dostoevsky

Epilepsy has been common throughout history, too. We learned in school about the work of famous people but never learned that many had epilepsy.

Up until the 1950s, epilepsy was something people rarely talked about. As a result, many people have hidden their epilepsy from the public. There were many great writers who may have had epilepsy, such as the poets Lord Byron and Edward Lear and novelists Feodor Dostoevsky and Gustave Flaubert. Some famous statesmen and leaders like Napoleon Bonaparte, Alexander the Great, Julius Caesar, and

Famous
people in
history who
had epilepsy

Peter the Great may also have had epilepsy. Socrates, the great Greek philosopher, and Pythagoras, Greek philosopher and mathematician, may well have had epilepsy. There is some evidence that epilepsy affected painter Vincent van Gogh, French patriot Joan of Arc, composer Peter Ilich Tchaikovsky, the apostle St. Paul, and Alfred Nobel, for whom the Nobel prize is named.

The achievements of these great people have shown us that epilepsy is not disabling — it is more common than you may think — and that people with epilepsy can lead productive lives.

What is epilepsy?

The word epilepsy comes from a Greek word that means "to possess, seize, or hold." In medicine, it describes short-lived bursts of uncontrolled energy in the brain. Epilepsy is common, affecting one in 150 to 200 people. One way to think about how many people have epilepsy is to imagine a football stadium full of people — 300 or 500 of them might have epilepsy.

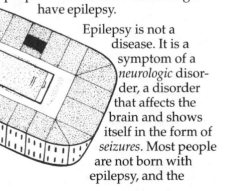

Epilepsy is not a disease. It is a symptom of a *neurologic* disorder, a disorder that affects the brain and shows itself in the form of *seizures*. Most people are not born with epilepsy, and the disorder is treatable in most cases. A seizure may strike anyone under certain conditions, for example, a brain infection or an allergic reaction to a drug. Seizures are more common among males, people under 20 years old, and senior citizens. Over half of the people who get epilepsy have their first seizure before age 15.

In many ways, the brain is like a computer — it even runs on electric currents. The electric signals in the brain are very small, but they are enough for one *neuron*, a type of nerve cell in the brain, to switch on another neuron. Epilepsy is a description of what happens when these cells "misfire." A seizure happens when a large group of neurons misfire — basically, a temporary "short circuit" of the brain.

The misfire may occur for different reasons. In patients with epilepsy, sometimes stress, not eating right, or lack of sleep may lead to a neuron misfire. At other times, the neuron misfire occurs because the brain has been hurt in an earlier accident or at birth. The hurt area of the brain interrupts the normal flow of cell firings. When routine firings are excessively altered, a seizure may happen.

Nerves throughout the body act like telephone lines, allowing the brain to send signals to the rest of the body. These lines are called the *central nervous system (CNS)* and the *peripheral nervous system (PNS)*. The CNS, includes the brain and spinal cord and is like an interstate highway. The PNS, made up of the nerves that sense and control movement, is like roads and lanes. Signals can travel down the CNS through the spinal cord until they reach their branch of the PNS. Then the signals go through the PNS to their particular nerve endings, say, in a toe or in an arm muscle.

The brain and its connections all over the body

What happens during a seizure

During a seizure, out-of-sync signals from the brain travel along the nervous system pathway to *sensors*, like the nerves that sense light in the eyes or the nerves that flex muscles. These out-of-sync signals may keep the brain from understanding what the eyes see, or may weaken leg-muscle tone and cause a person to lose balance and fall. This explains why people stare or why people fall down during a seizure. Some people lose consciousness entirely.

Other types of seizures

Aside from epilepsy, there are a number of conditions that can cause seizures. And treating some of these conditions requires a different kind of medical care than epilepsy treatment. That's why it's important that a doctor make a careful diagnosis.

Some seizures are caused by problems ranging from stroke to kidney or liver failure. Others are caused by withdrawal from (or allergic reactions to) drugs or alcohol. A small child may suffer a seizure because of a high fever. Doctors ask about head injuries their patients have had and might even test for a rare brain tumor. *Hypoglycemia,* also called low blood sugar, and severe infections of the brain can trigger seizures. Too low a level of minerals or vitamins in the bloodstream can trigger seizures too. In fact, the older people are when the first seizure occurs, the more likely there is a condition other than epilepsy.

Pseudoseizures

There are also conditions that look like seizures but really aren't seizures at all. They are called *pseudoseizures* — literally, false seizures. The main difference between true and false seizures is their source. Though a true seizure happens when nerves in the brain misfire without any clear cause, a pseudoseizure is a psychologic condition. Without really thinking about it, the mind "decides" to have a seizure.

Though pseudoseizures can look very much like true seizures, there are some physical differences between the two that can tip off a doctor to the correct diagnosis. For example, some people who have pseudoseizures stay conscious and even remember what happened during the event. They may act with a purpose or even violently. Pseudoseizures usually imitate generalized tonic–clonic seizures. In these seizures, the patient usually loses consciousness and has no memory of the event and can't act in a purposeful way.

Pseudoseizures are often a psychologic way of coping. They are a way in which the mind can try to deal with some difficulty. This means that proper treatment will be much different than for true seizures caused by epilepsy. This is why it is so important that patients do all they can to help their doctors make the correct diagnosis.

What causes epilepsy?

Epilepsy has many different causes. The cause for any one person may be difficult to figure out, because epilepsy is complex, and there is a lack of finely detailed medical knowledge about it. In 60% of all cases, no specific cause is found. These cases are called *idiopathic* or *cryptogenic* epilepsy and may be related to *genes* passed from parents to their children that make it more likely that the children will have seizures. Idiopathic epilepsy is usually detected early in life, often in people younger than 15 years old.

Although there is evidence that some kinds of epilepsy can be passed from parents to children, this does not happen very often. (A recent study found evidence that some people with epilepsy have abnormal genes on one of their sets of *chromosomes*.) According to the Epilepsy Foundation of America, even when both parents have epilepsy, the likelihood of passing epilepsy on to their child is about 10% to 12%. If only one parent has epilepsy, the chance drops to about 6%. Basically, unless both parents have a strong family history of epilepsy, the chances that any of their children will inherit the tendency to have seizures are very slight. Even so, if you have epilepsy and are planning to start a family, this is one more reason that you'll want to be sure to talk to a doctor.

There are other reasons why an infant may have epilepsy. Before birth, the baby could have had some sort of trouble, such as an infection, an injury to the head, or lack of oxygen. After they're born, babies are more susceptible to injury and some infections than are adults. By the age of 5 years, between 20% and 30% of people who will get epilepsy already have developed it.

Older children and adults are most likely to get epilepsy from head injuries. Injury is related to 40% of all epilepsy cases. This is one kind of epilepsy that is called *symptomatic*. Automobile accidents account for somewhere around 20,000 new cases of seizure disorders each year. Strokes or brain hemorrhages, because of their weakening effects, are a major source of symptomatic epilepsy and may account for as much as 50% of epileptic seizures in the elderly.

Diseases of the central nervous system or any condition that cuts the flow of blood to the brain can cause seizures. Diseases such as encephalitis and meningitis, as well as some poisons like lead and mercury, and drugs, like alcohol and cocaine, can cause seizures. These types of seizures may happen only once and may not be recurrent epilepsy.

Some cases of epilepsy can be avoided. Mothers should get proper medical and nutritional care before and during pregnancy. Proper care should continue once the baby is born. 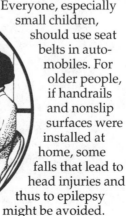 Everyone, especially small children, should use seat belts in automobiles. For older people, if handrails and nonslip surfaces were installed at home, some falls that lead to head injuries and thus to epilepsy might be avoided.

An accurate diagnosis of the cause of seizures is one of the first and most important steps that you can take in your health care. This is because different types of seizures are caused by different disorders. And different disorders need different medical treatments.

How doctors diagnose epilepsy

The first thing your doctor will want to find out is whether your symptoms represent seizures and whether they are caused by epilepsy or by something else. Your doctor will need a careful and thorough medical history — which requires your help.

The doctor will want to know such things as:

Questions your doctor will ask

- When did you have your first seizure?
- Did it happen after an injury?
- Were you tired, upset, or thirsty?
- Did you start, stop, or continue taking any medication just before the seizure?
- What happened when you had the seizure? (Give as much detail as possible.)
- Did you feel anything unusual or do anything special before the seizure started?
- How long did it last?
- How did you feel afterward?
- Did you have any memory of the seizure itself?
- Did you have any numbness or weakness afterward?
- Do seizures occur regularly, only in certain situations, at a certain time of day, at a regular time of the month (if you are a woman), or in any other pattern?

- Do seizures seem to come in groups, or do they happen one at a time?
- Does anyone else in your family have seizures of any sort?

The doctor probably also will want to talk with someone who has seen you have a seizure. This is because when you have a seizure you may have trouble remembering the details of exactly what happened. Questions this person might be asked about you are like the ones above, but they also may include:

- What kind of body movements did the patient make during the seizure?
- Did the patient collapse or remain sitting up or standing?
- Did the color of the patient's face change?
- Overall, how did the patient look?

Questions for your friend or family

You and your helper should take your time answering these and any other questions the doctor asks. Accuracy and details help the doctor make the right diagnosis. You may want to think about the questions above and talk about them with someone who has seen you have a seizure. This way, you'll be sure to remember all the details you possibly can. While you're at it, write everything down, and bring your notes when you see the doctor, so you don't forget to mention any details.

Tests

Neurologic tests that are part of most epilepsy physical exams check hearing, eye movement, swallowing, movements of muscles in the face, overall strength, reflexes, and coordination. A blood sample can be tested to measure levels of blood sugar, vitamins, minerals, and germs that cause infections.

Technology is very important in making the proper diagnosis, and there are a lot of tests and tools your doctor can use. Many of these tests measure electric activity in the brain — the *brain waves.*

The tests work because the brain uses small electric pulses to send instructions from one part of the brain to another and to and from nerves all over your body. These electric currents are very small, but sensitive medical equipment can find them through the skin. By understanding normal electric patterns in the brain and body, doctors and scientists can find patterns that are unusual, even the patterns of particular types of epilepsy.

EEG testing

One of the most important electronic tools for medicine is the *electroencephalograph (EEG)*. This device directly measures electric activity through small button-size sensors called *electrodes,* which are attached to the skin on a patient's head. Different patterns of activity from different spots on the scalp point to different kinds of epilepsy. The test is painless and harmless. The patient lies down during the test and may be asked to breathe quickly to hyperventilate (which can help make any unusual brain activity more noticeable to the machine).

Most normal waking EEG printouts show rapid, small changes in voltage throughout the brain. Tests done on people with epilepsy commonly show uneven activity or large changes in the voltage (spikes) of brain waves.

Sometimes, the brain functions perfectly normally during the test. And sometimes the electric patterns that the device is looking for happen too deep in the brain to be picked up by the EEG. When the EEG doesn't find anything unusual, it is common for the patient to get a continuous, 24-hour EEG monitoring, either during a hospital stay or at home. That way, the machine has a much better chance of picking up the telltale signals that doctors look for.

While the EEG is a very useful tool, it is not foolproof. About 5% of people without epilepsy have unusual EEG readings, and about 20% of people with epilepsy

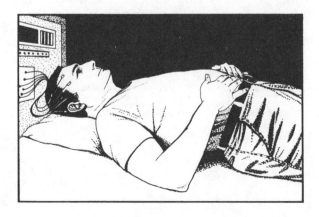

have normal EEGs. EEGs do not make a diagnosis of epilepsy unless a patient's medical history points to epileptic seizures too. EEGs can provide supportive evidence.

Other tests

Sometimes, the doctor will want to conduct more tests. One of these tests is the *computerized axial tomography (CAT or CT)* scan, which uses computer processing and x-ray beams to make a computer image of the brain. It's a large device used mostly in hospitals. The patient lies down on a movable table that slides into a hollowed-out machine. The CT scan looks at the brain from many positions, giving doctors a three-dimensional view of the brain.

A new device on the scene is the *magnetic resonance imager (MRI)*. All electric currents make magnetic fields, and the MRI measures the strength of these fields. Like a CT, an MRI gives a three-dimensional view of the brain. One advantage of MRI over CT is that it can "see" through the skull more clearly, and it can better define structures in the brain.

A *positron emission tomography (PET)* scan uses a safe, radioactive liquid, which is either injected or taken orally. The liquid gives off tiny particles called *positrons* that the PET scan detects. It maps how much energy different parts of the brain are using, and this can help find the area of the brain in which a seizure starts. This is not often used for epilepsy.

2 TYPES

To understand the differences among the types of seizures, you have to understand how the brain works. The brain is like a team of workers; each member has its own job to do, but each must communicate with the others. This means that specific parts of the brain are responsible for different duties. One part is in charge of understanding what the eyes see; another part directs speech; a different part controls the sense of smell. All the parts of the brain do their work and talk to each other over a network of cells called *neurons*. The neurons are the brain's telephone system, sending little electric charges from one point to another by either firing or not firing. This is how we think and move.

When a seizure occurs, the neurons are either firing when they shouldn't or not firing when they should. An uncontrolled discharge from neurons that affects several parts of deep regions and spreads to both sides of the brain is known as a generalized-onset seizure, a symptom of **generalized** epilepsy. If it occurs in only an isolated part of the brain, it is a partial seizure, a symptom of **focal** epilepsy.

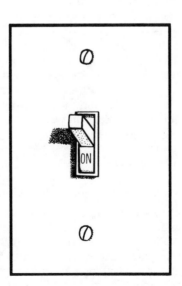

All epilepsies can be divided into these two categories.

It is important that your doctor figure out what form of epilepsy you have. Scientists have identified over 20 kinds of epileptic seizures. This *International Classification of Epileptic Seizures* helps doctors narrow down and finally pinpoint, as much as possible, the causes and treatments for each of the categories. Below is a discussion of some of these seizures.

Generalized-onset seizures

A **generalized-onset convulsive** seizure is what most people think of when they think about epilepsy. These seizures occur in 90% of all people with epilepsy, either as the only seizure or along with other seizures. The neurons' excess discharge may begin in one area, but it spreads throughout the brain. The term "generalized onset" refers to the fact that the entire brain is involved in the seizure, unlike in a partial seizure. These seizures cause muscle twitches, or convulsions; they may cause a person to grow rigid, salivate, urinate, or make other uncommon movements. This type of seizure may continue for 5 minutes or more. A person having a generalized-onset convulsive seizure will lose consciousness during the episode but will wake up shortly afterward. He or she will be unaware of having had a seizure but will feel tired and dazed.

Tonic–clonic, in past years called grand mal, seizures are a type of generalized-onset convulsive seizure. They occur when most of the neurons in the brain fire at the same time. (The seizure is *tonic* if the body stiffens, *clonic* if it jerks, or tonic-clonic if it stiffens, then jerks.) This usually involves convulsion, stiffening, jerking of the body, and loss of consciousness.

(But when only one part of the body is affected, it is focal epilepsy.)

In a generalized-onset **absence** seizure, also known in the past as a **petit mal** or **nonconvulsive** seizure, the part of the brain that keeps a person aware can't communicate with the brain cortex. The person may initially lose awareness for a few seconds but regains it. The person may lose muscle control and make repetitive motions, like chewing or fumbling with clothing. It may look like he or she has just "spaced out" for a moment. For children, this can lead teachers to suspect that the child just isn't paying attention in class.

Myoclonic seizures involve unusual neuron discharges in the *motor cortex* (a region of the brain that controls movement) and cause slight, involuntary jerking of the arms and legs, often early in the morning. Parents with myoclonic seizures may pass the tendency to myoclonic seizures on to their children. It is most common in young people, and for some

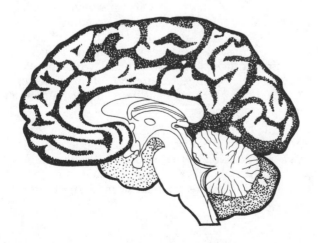

people it may be triggered by lack of sleep or too much alcohol. Many people have this disorder and don't know they have it. This is because it is often passed off as a "nervous tic." If they get medical treatment, though, most can expect significant improvement in their symptoms.

Other seizures are **atonic**, in which a person loses all muscle tone and falls. In a **tonic** seizure there is a sudden increase in muscle tone, or stiffening. **Clonic** seizures involve jerking of the body's muscles.

Status epilepticus is one seizure that lasts 30 minutes or more or a series of very closely spaced seizures. This is generally a medical emergency. (See page 27 for other important information on status epilepticus.)

Partial seizures

A **partial**, or focal, seizure takes place when an abnormal electric discharge occurs in only a small part of the brain (the *focus*). Other neurons prevent the excess discharge at the focus from spreading to other parts of the brain. If such a seizure occurs without a change of consciousness, it is **simple partial** (also sometimes called jacksonian or focal), while those seizures with a change, but not loss, of consciousness are called **complex partial** (also called psychomotor or temporal lobe).

A **simple partial** seizure generally lasts only a short time. In that time, the person having the seizure might smell an odd odor, feel a tingling, see flashing lights, jerk an arm or hand, or hear voices that he or she can't understand. The person remains conscious through this type of seizure.

2

If the electric discharge of a simple partial seizure covers a small area, the person may feel only a slight sensation but have no visible reaction. This sensation is an *aura* (see page 26). The aura often comes before a larger, convulsive seizure.

A person having a **complex partial** seizure may appear to be conscious but will lose contact with the outside world. The person may behave strangely at the beginning of the seizure — rubbing hands, fidgeting with an object, smacking lips, or grating teeth — this behavior is called an *automatism*. During the seizure some people may see or hear things that aren't there. Others remember events from the past. These seizures can vary in length from under a minute to around an hour. Afterward, the person may be confused and have a hard time talking with others. These seizures can become secondarily generalized.

Although there are many different kinds of seizures, they all have one thing in common — in most cases they can be controlled with medicine and other methods.

3   LIVING YOUR LIFE

"Talk with your doctor." That's always good advice when you have a health question, but for the treatment of epilepsy, it is extra important.

Be sure you understand and remember any instructions your doctor gives you. You might want to take notes during your appointments so you can be sure you don't forget any details. For example: How often should you take your medicine? How much should you take? What should you do if you forget to take a dose? Is there anything else you need to know?

But communication is much more than just understanding your doctor's instructions — it is also making sure you give your doctor any information that might be useful and asking any questions you have. After all, you want to know how to help yourself.

Don't be shy — ask your questions, even if you think they're not important. It's your doctor's job to help you understand. You probably will want to know how

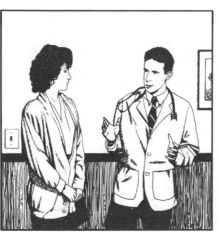

your medicine works. If you understand this, you can get a better feel for why it is so important that you stick to your medication schedule. Also, if you know how your medicine works, you may be able to spot side effects more easily. Remember, your doctor will want to know about any side effects you have.

The doctor gives you a lot of important information, but you have to give him or her important information too. Keep track of when you have seizures. Have you noticed any side effects? Have you been tired or had headaches? If you have a "funny feeling that something isn't right," try to explain the feeling to your doctor.

The information you give your doctor will help him or her fine-tune your medication schedule. Maybe the amount of medicine you take needs to be changed — *but only if your doctor says so!* Maybe you need a different medicine. Only your doctor can know these things and only if you give all the information you can.

Good communication leads to good medicine and good control. If you have tried to talk with your doctor and don't feel you are getting useful answers, talk over your concerns with your doctor. *Remember:* Your health is the reason you see a doctor; get the service you deserve.

Antiepileptic drugs

A class of drugs called *antiepileptic drugs,* or anticonvulsants, is given by doctors to treat epilepsy. These drugs are taken every day, sometimes several times a day, for many years. The drugs do not cure epilepsy, but they help control the seizures.

Careful testing is done to find the cause and type of a person's seizures, because different types of seizures are best treated by different kinds of antiepileptic drugs. The following is a list of common antiepileptic medications.

Proper medication

All anticonvulsant drugs have been associated with side effects. Talk with your physician if you have any questions on side effects.

This is a list of some of the most common drugs. They are listed by their chemical names, and a common brand name is in the parentheses.

Carbamazepine (Tegretol®)

Clonazepam (Klonopin®)

Ethosuximide (Zarontin®)

Phenobarbital (No most common brand name)

Phenytoin (Dilantin®)

Primidone (Mysoline®)

Valproic acid (Depakene®)

Divalproex sodium (Depakote®)

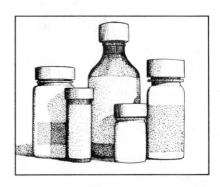

Surgery

Surgery can help only certain people. It should be considered in a limited group of those who have epilepsy. Surgery as a treatment of epilepsy involves removing the part of the brain that is the focus of seizures. Surgery is used only in cases in which either the seizures or the amount of medication required to control them would disable the patient. The seizures must be limited to a very small part of the brain to allow surgeons to remove the part, and it must be a part of the brain that would not leave the patient impaired if it was removed. As a result, surgery as treatment is used as a last resort, only after other options have been tried. For patients who are surgical candidates, surgery generally stops seizures for at least 5 years (with or without drugs or auras) in 55% to 70% of cases.

Help yourself and tell others

Let others know about your epilepsy. You need to open up to people around you. Not only are there things that others can do to help you if you have a seizure, there are myths that many people don't know are untrue and, sometimes, these myths may even be dangerous to you.

Myth: A person having a seizure can swallow his or her tongue.

Fact: It is physically impossible to swallow your tongue. But people who don't know this might try to force the mouth open, and that can injure the mouth and teeth.

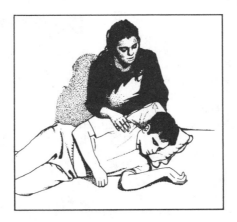

3

What is true is that the tongue might block the airway in the mouth — but the best way to prevent this is to turn the person having a seizure on his or her side. Then the tongue will fall to the side of the mouth, leaving the airway clear for normal breathing. Artificial respiration should be tried *only* if the person does not start breathing again after the seizure stops.

Myth: A person having a seizure needs to be held down.

Fact: Again, this myth can cause injury. Instead, helpers should move sharp or hard objects out of the way and try to place something soft, like a pillow or a rolled-up jacket, under the person's head. Also, remove eyeglasses and loosen collars and ties to help prevent injury.

Myth: All seizures require quick medical attention, maybe an ambulance, too.

Fact: Generally, only seizures that last longer than about 5 to 10 minutes, or a series of seizures, one right after another, require emergency medical attention. Many ambulance trips (as well as a lot of money) are wasted on unnecessary calls. You and your doctor can talk about what *you* need.

Myth: There is a way to help a person having a seizure "snap out of it."

Fact: There is usually nothing anyone can do to end a seizure. It's best just to stay with the person during the seizure and be supportive and reassuring when he or she regains consciousness. Some people may be confused and disoriented — they may appreciate someone calling a taxi, relative, or friend to pick them up or offering to walk with them to their destination.

Whom should you tell?

Whom should you tell about your epilepsy? Family, friends, coworkers, teachers — these are all people you should think about talking to. If your seizures are under good control, you may want to tell only your family and closest friends. But if your control isn't perfect, you'll want to dispel the myths listed above for people who might be around if you have a seizure. They'll feel more confident, and they'll be in a better position to help you.

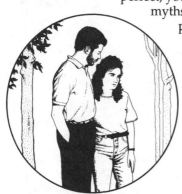

Sometimes people might react negatively when you tell them, but their reaction is probably the result of just the kind of misunderstanding that you're clearing up. After all, you're just as much of a person as anyone else, just like the other millions of people in the United States who have epilepsy. And if people you tell still let their emotions block their understanding, keep your sense of humor and don't take it to heart. Most times, though, you'll probably find that people want to learn more and be helpful.

Should you tell a date or new boss? It's a tricky question. On one hand, it's better to tell someone before you have a seizure so they will be prepared. On the other hand, it's easier to tell somebody if you know them pretty well. One thing epilepsy isn't is a "deep, dark secret." It's just another part of you. So maybe you won't want to mention epilepsy to your blind date, but after a while, when it feels right, you may want to talk about it.

Triggers

Epilepsy is unpredictable. A seizure can happen at just about any time — that's why it is so important to take your medicine consistently. The correct dose of medicine in your bloodstream is the number-one priority for preventing seizures. But there are certain situations that, for some people, can increase the likelihood of a seizure. If you know what these situations are, you can avoid them and reduce the chance of having a seizure.

Stress

Stress can be one of these factors. Everybody has stress, but too much stress and changes in the body it causes can help bring on seizures. A single stressful moment causes the release of the hormone *adrenaline*.

This hormone can increase blood circulation and breathing rate.

It would be great to avoid stress in the first place, but when you can't, stress-reduction techniques may help prevent some seizures. The next time you are feeling "all stressed out," try this simple exercise: Close your eyes. Slow down your breathing. Every time you breathe out, count down a number from ten to one. With each number, try to "feel" your muscles getting more relaxed. By the time you get to "one," you'll probably feel a whole lot better. The thing that made you tense will still be there, but you'll be in a better frame of mind to deal with it. There are many other methods of dealing with stress, some of which may work even better for you.

You have to be sure to get enough rest, too. Too little sleep, or irregular sleep, can cause more frequent seizures. If you just can't get to sleep, try a relaxation technique, such as the one above.

Sleep

Also, eat properly. Your parents were right when they said you need to eat well-balanced meals to maintain your health.

For a few people, flickering lights and sounds can be triggers for seizures. Two of the most common sources of flickering lights are television and video games. Several years ago, a popular music video that had rapidly changing images was banned in Britain because of the number of seizures it was causing. If flickers affect you, you'll probably want to avoid these sources. Another problem might be caused by shadow and light outdoors. Sunglasses may help.

Flickering lights

Auras

You may have an "early warning system" for seizures. Some people, just before a convulsive seizure, sense an aura. An aura is a strange sensation or feeling. It might be a buzzing in the ear, dizziness, sickness to the stomach, or a powerful emotion. In fact, just about any sensation, if it regularly occurs just before a seizure, can be an aura. You can use auras. If you sense that you are about to have a seizure, you can take quick precautions to ensure your safety. Auras themselves are actually simple partial seizures.

Just because you haven't noticed an aura doesn't mean you don't have them; many people don't notice them until they've done a little research. Here's how to do it. After you've had a seizure, try to remember if you noticed anything unusual just before the seizure — even an unexplained feeling of fear can be an aura — and write it down. If, after a while, you notice a pattern, you may have found an aura.

Take an active role

For your epilepsy treatment to work best, *you* have to take an active role. That means making sure to take your medicine on schedule, knowing what others should do if you have a seizure and telling them, and eating right. Learn as much as you can about the condition so you can be "tuned in" and notice side effects or be aware of situations you might otherwise take for granted. The more you know, the less uncertainty can stop you from living life to its fullest.

Take your medication. It's obvious that medicine your doctor prescribes will help you, but it may not be so obvious how important it is that you carefully follow your medical schedule. For medicine to do its job, it has to be at a fairly constant level in the blood. At the right level, it helps block the out-of-sync signals in the brain from triggering other cells to fire. But your body uses up medicine a little at a time, something like the way it uses air — you need a constant supply of both medicine and air. If the medicine level drops too low, it cannot serve its function. If it's too high, you can have unwanted side effects. A regular schedule, though, makes sure that you always have the right medicine levels. (See page 37 for tips that help you remember to take your medicine.)

Be consistent. Your best tool for taking your medicine on time is habit. Take your medicine at the same time every day. You can even count out pills for the day each morning. Then, with a glance, you can be sure you did (or didn't) take a particular dose. And let habit work for you so you can be sure you don't run out of your medicine. Get your prescription refilled regularly.

A very important note: If you don't follow your doctor's advice about how much medicine to take and when to take it, you run the risk of having a seizure. A serious medical complication of seizures is *status epilepticus*. Status epilepticus is a prolonged seizure that lasts 30 minutes or more or a series of short seizures, one right after another, where the patient doesn't regain consciousness between seizures. It is usually a medical emergency, and it always requires a doctor's help. Some people with epilepsy may have this condition at one time or another. The good news is that the best way to prevent status epilepticus is to keep on the medical schedule your doctor recommends.

Store medication properly. You also want to be sure that your medicine is full strength. That means you have to be careful about how you store it. Generally, medicine should be stored in a dark, cool, dry place — exactly the opposite of a warm, humid bathroom medicine cabinet.

Know what you're mixing. Be aware that mixing drugs — whether they are epilepsy medicine, alcohol, aspirin, birth-control pills, antibiotics, or anything else — can cause unexpected results. That's why you want your doctor to know about any other medicines you are taking. If your epilepsy medicine doesn't work well with other medicine you are taking for another problem, it doesn't mean you can't relieve the other problem. Your doctor can tell you what you can substitute or whether you should simply change the amount of the other medicine you take.

Alcohol

Alcohol is classified as a depressant drug. That means it can slow your body down, as well as possibly make you feel down. Many antiepileptic drugs increase this effect. So, together, they can have a big effect on you. That's why you should talk to your doctor about your drinking "limit."

Birth-control pills

Birth-control pills may be less effective when a woman takes some antiepileptic medicines. So, if you take birth-control pills, be sure the doctor who is treating you for epilepsy knows you take them.

Antibiotics

Some antibiotics, which doctors use to treat a wide variety of infections, can suddenly raise or lower the amount of antiepileptic medicine in your system. Be sure your doctor knows if you are taking both.

Emergency situations. In an emergency, you may not be able to tell people about your epilepsy. So it's a good idea to carry identification. Keep a piece of paper with you that lists all your medicines and the fact that you have epilepsy. It can help doctors be sure that epilepsy doesn't become a complication. Also, emergency workers are trained to look for Medic-Alert ID bracelets. If you wear one, they'll spot it fast. During a seizure, it will help concerned people help you. For more information about the bracelet, call Medic-Alert at (800) ID-ALERT.

Support systems

You also will want to seek support from others. (See page 39 for information on support groups.) A supportive environment is good for your well-being. Take full advantage of available support systems; social workers, counselors, psychologists, and other health care workers can be very helpful. A supportive (and informed) friend or spouse is extremely helpful; his or her presence before and after a seizure will be a

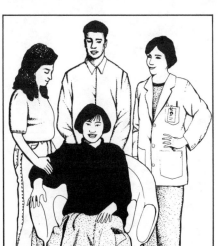

great source of support. Family support is essential. Be aware of the concerns epilepsy places on them, too.

But the support others offer can't help you much if you don't accept your epilepsy.

Sometimes people may want to extend special privileges to you. It's tempting to take these offers, but they can backfire by making you (and them) think that you really are different. It's a lot easier to feel happy about yourself when you feel you're in control and you don't have to rely on others so much. (But remember, only hermits don't rely on anyone ever!) This doesn't mean you should participate in unsafe activities, but it does mean you don't want to be treated as less than capable.

4 USEFUL POINTS

Safety

Safety is an important consideration for everyone, including people with epilepsy. But safety considerations don't have to stop many people from doing just about anything they want to do — if they follow a few common-sense guidelines.

Safety starts in the home. Epilepsy doesn't have to change your life a whole lot, but if you live alone or if your seizures aren't under good control, you may want to make minor changes. In the kitchen, you may want to use a microwave oven more often than an open range to reduce the risk of burns from an exposed heat source. In the bathroom, shallow baths and showers can reduce the risk of drowning. The bathroom should have a door that opens outward so if someone inside collapses against the door, someone trying to help can open the door and reach them. Extrawide beds and futons (a kind of mattress placed on or near the floor) can reduce the risk of falling out of bed. Some people's doctors advise them to purchase safety pillows, which reduce the risk of suffocation during sleep.

Transportation

Our society puts a lot of emphasis on driving cars. In some places, it can be inconvenient to get where you want to without a car, and many folks think that people with epilepsy can't get a driver's license. But people whose epilepsy is under control (as defined by the state they live in) can get a driver's license. In fact, some groups of people with epilepsy have lower accident rates than some groups of people who don't have epilepsy.

Some states have time periods for which a person must be seizure free, usually 3 months to a year. Other states have no specific waiting period and decide on a person-by-person basis. In some states, a physician is required to report seizures. A physician's recommendation can shorten the period in some states. You'll probably need a letter from your doctor in just about any case. All in all, the trend seems to be toward fewer restrictions. You should check with your local motor vehicle agency for further details. Also, check with your doctor.

And don't forget auto insurance, though it may be difficult to get. Some states have started pool auto insurance plans. Groups of companies, and sometimes states themselves, underwrite these plans, which guarantee insurance for all drivers.

But you have to be realistic and honest; a driver who has a seizure places himself or herself, as well as others, at risk of serious injury. So if you can't drive, or if you're still in your waiting period, here are some suggestions that will help you get around:

- It may seem obvious, but if there's a good public-transportation system where you live, use it. At first, it might seem hard to find out about maps, timetables, and transfers, but you'll probably be riding like a pro in no time.
- Try a car pool. That doesn't mean you have to drive; you'll just help pay for gas and tolls. Anyhow, many people are glad to have the company while they commute to work or go shopping.
- There may be someone in your neighborhood who would like to make a little extra money as your personal "taxi driver." Students, homemakers, and retirees are good people to

try. If you don't know the person, you'll probably want to ask for a few references.
• Check with your local chapter of the Epilepsy Foundation of America (see page 39); they may know of other services you can use.

Sports and other activities

Many people worry that epilepsy can make partici-pating in sports unwise. The truth, however, is that almost anyone whose seizures are under control and who wants to participate in sports can. But before you start, check with your doctor. He or she will tell you whether the sport you've chosen is okay in your case. For example, boxing (where head injuries are com-mon) and sports involving dangerous heights are probably not a good idea. You may be given special instructions, such as the tips below, about the safest way to participate in the sport you are interested in.

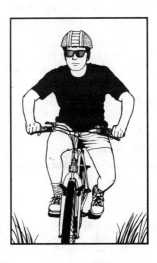

• *In general:* If you feel unusually tired or have missed your medicine, you may not want to participate that day.
• *Bicycling.* It surprises many people that bicycling can be safe for people

with epilepsy. You don't want to ride on busy streets (because of the danger from traffic), and you do want to ride with a friend who knows what to do if you have a seizure. Wear a helmet, and perhaps elbow and knee pads, and you can have fun as well as safe exercise.

- *Swimming.* If seizure control is very good, it may be safe to swim with someone — but avoid swimming alone. It's a good idea if your swimming partner is strong enough to come to your aid if you do have a seizure in the water. He or she will keep your head above water and get you to land. And, of course, be cautious, and think safety.

Some people worry that exercise will bring on a seizure, but, in fact, the chance that this will happen is very slight. The Epilepsy Foundation of America says, "In most cases, persons with epilepsy can take part in sports or other vigorous activities, although a lot depends on the degree of seizure control, the type of sport, and the physician's recommendation."

Children probably will want to participate in gym class at school. It helps them develop confidence in themselves. But if the doctor advises against gym class, try to explain to your child why he or she can't join in. Disappointment isn't always so bad when the child understands the reason. (You may need to talk to your child's teachers, too. See page 50.)

Talk to your doctor about situations to avoid.

Memory tricks

Some people seem to be able to remember anything and everything. Unfortunately, not all of us are so gifted. People with epilepsy have something especially important to remember: to take their medicine on time. In fact, epilepsy itself can make it harder to remember things.

Many types of seizures and medications affect the memories of people with epilepsy. When you have a seizure, it blocks your memory, sometimes not allowing you to remember anything that occurred during the seizure or the seizure itself. Also, some medicines can make it a bit harder to remember things. The following tips and tricks will help anyone remember more things more clearly and more accurately.

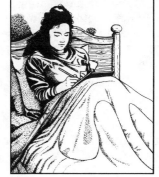

Write things down: If you put something important down on paper, you don't have to remember it. That's why some people make a point each morning of listing all the things they want to do during the day. Then, as the day goes on, they cross off the items they've done and look to see what else they need to do. Other people like to take time at the end of the day to list the things they want to do the next day. It doesn't matter when you make a list, but if you make it the same time each day, you won't forget to make the list itself.

You also may want to keep a pen and paper with you. That way, if you are talking on the phone and hear something you want to remember, or if your doctor has instructions for you, you'll be able to write these things down. (Some of these things will wind up on your next daily list, too.) Don't be shy about taking notes when someone is talking to you; they'll probably be happy that you think what they are saying is important enough for you to make the effort. Also, calendars make it easy to remember appointments.

Another benefit of writing something down is that, in a sense, you repeat everything to yourself. And repetition is a good way to help remember things.

Make it a habit: Humans are creatures of habit, and you can use this to your advantage. If you always put on a hat when you go outside, get in the habit of putting it on only after you've locked the door. Then, if you're outside wearing your hat, you won't have to wonder whether you remembered to lock the door. It's easy to remember to use dental floss every day if you're in the habit of using it every time you brush your teeth.

Make it stand out: Sometimes it's hard to remember if you've locked your front door or turned off the upstairs hall light. Next time, do something unusual as you turn off that light — whistle a funny song, or turn the switch off with your left hand (if you're right handed). Doing two things at once or one thing in an unusual way creates a thought connection in your mind. So if you remember whistling the funny song, you'll know you turned the light off.

Rhyme: Before people invented writing, cultures kept their histories as long, memorized stories. And one of the most important tricks the storytellers used was rhyme. Rhyme makes it easier to remember two things, or words, if you are only sure of one. School teachers use this when they teach youngsters to help them remember spelling rules, like "I before E, except after C," or the days of months, "Thirty days hath

September, April, June, and November." Silly rhymes are sometimes even easier to remember.

Acronyms: Not many people would remember the official name of the National Aeronautics and Space Administration, but it's easy to remember "NASA." And how many phone numbers have you seen where a company has spelled out a word with the numbers? It's just a way to make the number easier to remember. You can make up acronyms, too — like "WOW" for Wilbur and Orville Wright, the Wright brothers.

Special tips to help you remember medication: Pill boxes, the kind with separate compartments for each day of the week, can be a big help. At the beginning of the week, count out all of your medicine for the next 7 days. This helps you keep track of pills you've taken and the ones you haven't. For example, if you take medicine four times a day and you have two pills left, it's a snap to figure out whether you took your second dose.

It can be hard for people on the go to maintain a routine. But a watch with an alarm can remind you that it's time for your next dose. Just set the alarm to go off when it's time to take your medicine. And those new electronic pocket organizers can even display a message that reminds you why you set the alarm in the first place.

Mood changes

Seizures and the medicine people with epilepsy take to control them can affect mood. Because people with epilepsy can never be sure of when or where a seizure will happen, many of these people feel anxiety. High anxiety levels will not only increase the chance of having a seizure but also can affect how people act in social and work situations.

Anxiety is basically a feeling of loss of control. If a person feels a regaining of control, he or she may be able to reduce the anxiety. Knowing what causes seizures and how to avoid the causes are one way to regain control. If you recognize an aura, that's even better. Another way is not to hide epilepsy from friends, family, and coworkers, so that they'll know what to do if you have a seizure. People relax when they know they aren't trying to conceal their condition.

Relaxing and using relaxation techniques is another important step toward reducing anxiety. But relaxation does not mean doing nothing. Activity can be relaxing, and a person can be inactive but still feel a lot of anxiety. By learning to relax, a person can learn to spot the early signs of anxiety and perhaps identify a link between seizures and anxiety.

Feeling down is also a problem for some people. Everybody feels down once in a while, but sometimes the feeling can seem like a big burden. These people may lose their appetites or just have no energy. For some, epilepsy brings on feelings of guilt or "not feeling good enough." These people lose a lot of their self-worth. Most often they do not even realize they are depressed; instead, friends and loved ones notice the condition. There are several remedies and activities that help combat depression, such as talking to someone, writing letters, going for walks, helping other people, and seeing friends.

Support groups

Support groups and family can help with these feelings; most epilepsy groups are open and sponsored by sympathetic organizations. Doctors recommend these groups because they know that getting answers to your questions is nothing to be shy about. After all, the more you understand, the better you can adjust your lifestyle to get the most out of life. And the more people feel in control of their lives, the more they are confident and happy.

There are a number of formal organizations you can turn to for information and discussion about epilepsy. The biggest one is The Epilepsy Foundation of America (EFA). The EFA's national office is at 4351 Garden City Drive, Landover, MD 20785. Its local phone number is (301) 459-3700.

Epilepsy Foundation of America

The Epilepsy Foundation of America has local affiliates throughout the country. The toll-free phone number, (800) EFA-1000, is open for referrals and answers to questions between 9 AM and 6 PM eastern time. They also provide information, job placement, training, and advocacy programs, in addition to sponsoring medical research.

The Epilepsy Foundation of America also has the world's most complete library on epilepsy. The library's toll-free phone number is (800) EFA-4050.

Professional counselors can help people with epilepsy and their families understand and deal with epilepsy. Counselors can often help you when you have trouble with practical matters, like finding a job or getting insurance.

Other support groups provide much information and moral support. These groups are gatherings of people with epilepsy who share tips, triumphs, and problems with other members of the group. It can be a real comfort to see that other people have concerns that are similar to yours — you are not alone.

Your doctor might know about support groups in the area. For children there are epilepsy support camps. Support groups work best when everyone tries to have a positive, helpful attitude. If the first group you go to has too many complainers who are not interested in dealing better with life, find another group.

If there is no convenient support group in your area, you can form your own. But forming your own group takes a little preparation. Here are some ideas:

- Remember that, at first, some people may be shy about discussing their epilepsy.
- Write a short handout that describes what your group would do and lists you as the contact person, and ask your doctor if he or she will give the handout to other patients with epilepsy.
- Organize a lecture about epilepsy. Maybe your doctor will speak or recommend someone else who can. Greet people at the door with your handout. (And if you are going to advertise the lecture in a local newspaper, you may get the ad fee reduced if you call the paper well before you want the ad to run.)

Once you get the group going, try these tips:

- See if a school, club, or church will let you use a room for free to have your meetings. If you can make the meetings the same time and place, it's easier for members of your group to remember when and where to come. Also, you can take turns bringing refreshments, if you want.

- Invite a doctor to some or all of your meetings. This way, you'll know that you are sharing accurate medical information. And, of course, a doctor can answer questions.
- Don't forget to keep trying to attract new members. New people can bring new ideas and perspectives into your group.

4

5 FINANCIAL

It's important to know your rights as a person with epilepsy. Job hunting is hard enough without having to deal with misunderstandings about epilepsy. Discrimination based on people not knowing about epilepsy can be a problem, whether you're applying for a job, health insurance, or auto insurance. By knowing your rights, though, you can search for a job or insurance with confidence.

Many mistaken ideas and beliefs have kept people with epilepsy from having the jobs they really want. One common myth is that computer monitors trigger seizures, when, in fact, there are only a few people with photosensitive epilepsy, which makes a person sensitive to flickering lights.

One important resource for job placement is The Epilepsy Foundation of America's Training and Placement Service (TAPS), a nationwide program aimed at helping find job opportunities for people with epilepsy.

Your local chapter of the EFA can inform you about your state's laws on discrimination at work. If your state has a human or civil rights commission or a protection and advocacy agency, it may be helpful too.

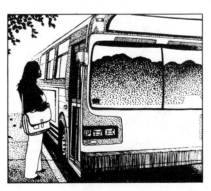

Jobs

Some things to keep in mind while job hunting:

- Learn about the job you are applying for
  before you interview. Pay close attention to
  what the work requires. You probably
  shouldn't be applying for a position where
  having a seizure would be dangerous, such as
  in a job where you would be working in high,
  open places.
- Take action if you believe you were discrimi-
  nated against. For example, if you are turned
  down because of your medical condition for a
  job in which your condition would pose no
  danger or disability, and you otherwise fully
  qualify, bring the matter to the attention of the
  appropriate authorities, such as your local
  health department, the Department of Labor,
  and advocacy groups for the disabled.

Discrimination

When you look for employment, questions about
health are usually asked of people with obvious
disabilities, not people with epilepsy. But questions do
come up, whether on an application or in an interview. The recently enacted Americans With Disabilities Act (ADA) prohibits private employers from
discriminating against persons with disabilities with
respect to any term or condition of employment.
Specifically, the ADA makes it illegal for private
employers with more than 15 employees to discrimi-
nate against "qualified individuals with disabilities"
and requires such employers to provide "reasonable
accommodations" for disabled workers, unless the
employer can show that it would be an "undue
hardship" to do so. While the employment provisions
of the ADA apply only to private employers, the

5

Federal Rehabilitation Act of 1973 imposes similar requirements on federal agencies, companies that have contracts with the federal government, and companies that receive federal financial assistance.

Health insurance

Some medical insurance companies either penalize people with epilepsy or won't insure them at all. Many companies offer limited coverage, usually excluding epilepsy-related expenses. In an age when medical costs have skyrocketed and you have to have insurance to get into some hospital emergency rooms, the availability of Medicare, Medicaid, or comparable coverage is very important.

Group insurance plans provided by employers can be an excellent way to get health insurance for people with epilepsy and their families. The plans tend to have less selective requirements than private plans.

Another option is a plan that covers you only for injury or accidental death. Many such policies do not require a medical history or examination. But when you look into these policies, make sure that accidents resulting from preexisting conditions are not excluded.

Some employers will not hire people with epilepsy because these workers are considered accident prone and will cause the company's liability insurance premiums to go up. Others think that an employee with epilepsy cannot get worker's compensation. This often causes people with epilepsy to hide their condition. In one study, 50% of employees had not told their employers about their epilepsy at the time they started their jobs. If you or a potential employer has questions about insurance, contact your state's insurance commission.

But the truth is that people with epilepsy are more reliable than other people about attendance and job performance. On average, someone who has occasional seizures misses only 1 work hour out of every 1,000. (That's just 1 day every 4 years.)

There are many other factors that determine a person's qualifications for a job, and these should be weighed just as much as any medical condition. Past academic and work experience and a person's abilities should be the major considerations.

If you are eligible as a low-income candidate or are unable to find private insurance, apply to the federally funded Medicare and Medicaid programs.

Income assistance

If your epilepsy does reduce your ability to work, then you may qualify for Supplementary Security Income, or SSI, under the Social Security Administration (SSA). The SSI program is designed to help people who have small incomes because they are unable to work or can work only a little. The eligibility requirements are complicated, but if you can show the SSA that your epilepsy hurts your ability to work, you may be able to get some assistance.

Children who will be receiving benefits do not have to show they cannot work, of course, but you do have to show they cannot thrive the way other children can. This should be noted in the application for benefits, because it could make a difference in their eligibility.

If you are thinking of looking for a job after you apply for some kind of unemployment or disability benefits, you probably want to start getting your benefits first, before you look for a job. It is easier to get back into the SSA system if a job does not work out than it is to try to get benefits after you have already been working.

When applying for any SSA-sponsored program, keep a few things in mind:

Social Security application tips

- Apply early. The sooner you apply to Social Security, the sooner you'll receive your benefits. Even if you don't think you'll be eligible, apply anyway. As an added incentive to apply early, medical assistance program coverage begins at the time you apply, if you are accepted.

- Although the SSA runs both programs, SSI and medical assistance require separate applications and have different review processes. Apply for both at the same time — don't wait for the SSI's approval before you file for medical assistance.

- Remember that the key to winning approval is to show clearly the relationship between epilepsy and your ability to do the task required of a job. Eligibility for benefits depends on your ability to work.

- Your doctor can help you with the application. According to the Epilepsy Foundation of America, the SSA classifies seizures in a different way from the one doctors use. Before your doctor gives your records to the SSA, ask him or her to make the report according to the classifications the SSA uses. How often seizures happen is a major consideration for benefits. Since having a seizure can often mean wiping out your memory of having had it, you should ask your family, friends, coworkers, and other witnesses to recall any seizures you don't remember having.

- If you are turned down, appeal the decision. The SSA has been known to deny some applications incorrectly.

Whether applying for a job or for health or auto insurance, it's best to be up front about your epilepsy. Often, a lifetime of hiding the condition makes it easy to forget to tell insurers or to underestimate the frequency or severity of seizures. All medical problems should be listed if they make a difference in your ability to work. For example, the effects of any medication, social or emotional adjustment, or even a learning disorder should be listed.

It's important to be open about your epilepsy. People fear what they don't know. Learn as much as you can about your condition. If you can speak knowledgeably and confidently about your epilepsy, chances are your confidence can rub off on potential employers or insurers and set their minds at ease.

Remember, the key to getting insurance and employment is to know your rights, know about your condition, shop around, and look into all the options available.

6   RAISING A FAMILY

Having a baby
Epilepsy does not have to have too big an effect on your lifestyle, including parenthood. When mother and child get proper care, women with epilepsy usually have healthy babies after uncomplicated pregnancies. But make no mistake, pregnancies can be tricky, and you'll have to be in close touch with your doctor. If you are on medication and are thinking about pregnancy, consult your physician immediately. And if you are pregnant now, call your doctor today (if you haven't already).

Seizures in pregnant women can be a problem, particularly for the fetus. Repeated generalized seizures may deprive the unborn child of oxygen or injure it if the mother falls during a seizure. In mothers with epilepsy who are treated with antiepileptic drugs, the incidence of birth defects is two to three times greater than that of mothers without epilepsy. In general, about 90% of women with epilepsy who receive antiepileptic drugs during pregnancy will deliver normal children free of birth defects. Most medicine-related birth defects happen in the first three

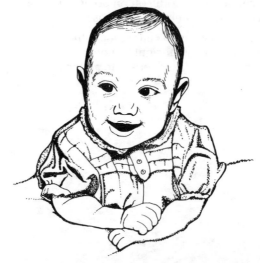

months of pregnancy, so it is very important to talk to a doctor early, before getting pregnant. This is even more important for women who are taking two drugs to control their epilepsy. The doctor might need to make adjustments in the woman's treatment.

If you plan on breast-feeding, it is important to discuss this with your doctor.

But antiepileptic drugs are important for mothers-to-be. A seizure is likely to be more dangerous to the baby. Seizures can upset blood flow to the fetus. And if the mother falls during a seizure because medical control has been reduced, it is possible that the fetus will be injured. *So don't change your medication schedule during pregnancy unless your doctor says to.*

Parenthood can be tough on a person with epilepsy. Seizures due to sleep loss when attending to the baby at night may be common, so parents should take care to get enough sleep. Parents also should try to feed their infants while sitting down, a precaution to keep the child safe if they have a sudden seizure. Similar safeguards should be taken when the parent is alone with the child to minimize injury to the infant. You can change diapers on the floor instead of the table, and baths should be shallow. In order to avoid radical changes in lifestyle, activities could be shared with the other partner so two people are present.

Lack of sleep and parenting tips

Talking to kids

Some people don't want to talk to their children about epilepsy, because they worry their children will react negatively. It turns out, though, that children who learn about epilepsy before they see a seizure are generally very supportive and want to do whatever they can to help Mom or Dad.

Parents also should be careful about keeping their pills out of a child's reach (children like to imitate their parents and may try to take medicine, too). As the child grows, make him or her aware of epilepsy and what he or she should do during a seizure.

When your child has epilepsy

It is extremely important that someone with epilepsy gets proper care and support. Treating children differently or treating them as impaired during the growing years could have lasting negative effects. A school-age child is under great social pressure from other children; parents should make sure that the child participates in as many activities as his or her condition allows. Parents should be sure that their children can explain epilepsy to their friends in a positive, educational way, and parents also should be aware of any teasing that may go on. Children tend to hide teasing and deny that it's a problem. But teasing can cause them to lose confidence in social situations.

A young person's fear of having a seizure in public may cause him or her to withdraw socially and not participate in activities with other people. Children need to be encouraged to be open with their friends about their condition. Hiding it or withdrawing because of it only creates a burden for a child who has epilepsy.

Talk with teachers and baby-sitters

If you are the parent of a child with epilepsy, it is important to talk to the child's teachers and baby-sitters. Many teachers don't know what they should do to help a child having a seizure. A discussion with your child's teachers can clear things up and put them completely at ease. Also, teachers can help ensure that your child always takes his or her medicine, and they can be on the lookout for any school activities, like shop, where your child might want to be extra careful.

Adolescence

Adolescence can be a difficult time for both parents and children with epilepsy. Children want to try their wings, and parents have to learn how to adjust. It is a time of increased social pressures for children, and they may be tempted to be more concerned about joining in than in using common sense. Adolescence is a normal part of growing up, but it can have negative effects on epilepsy control.

Sometimes, as a way of showing their independence, teens will become lazy about taking their antiepileptic medicine, and they might even skip it from time to time. This is obviously a bad idea, but a child may feel that parents' warnings and advice are just nagging. Teens are more open to advice when they don't think that parents are trying to run their lives. It's also a good idea to be sure that teens understand as much as possible about epilepsy, and that being seizure free for a while does not mean that they can stop taking their medicine. Understanding is a great motivator. For other ideas, talk to your child's doctor or contact the EFA.

Another possible problem is illegal drugs and alcohol. (See pages 7 and 28.) These can make it hard to keep good seizure control. Again, one of the best ways to keep teens from dangerous experimentation is to be sure they know all they can about epilepsy and control.

School

School can be a big worry for the parents of a child with epilepsy. Whether the student is about to start preschool or college, parents worry because they can't be there to guide their children. But parents *can* work with their children to help them take better care of themselves.

Epilepsy should not stand in the way of an education. Nor should the condition affect the quality of a student's education. A little planning can make school easier.

Teachers should know if a student has epilepsy. They can be helpful if the child has a seizure; they can calm and teach other children about epilepsy; and they will better understand how to help if the child needs help with his or her lessons.

The idea that epilepsy makes one person any different from any other person is largely a myth, yet there are still misunderstandings about epilepsy. Some children with epilepsy have trouble learning in a few areas, such as understanding

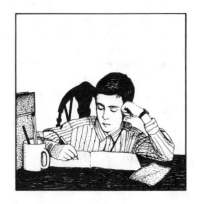

spatial relationships, recognizing visual images, learning different languages, or memorizing things. For many of these children, school is the first time they realize their 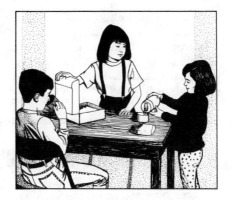 limitations, and they can feel discouraged. Some become disinterested, frustrated, embarrassed, or angry, and a few will give up trying to learn. But children who have epilepsy can adapt to limitations just as easily as other children who are weak in one area but excel in another.

Sometimes a teacher will tell parents their child is inattentive in class, stares out a window, or nods off to sleep. That's because many kinds of medicine for epilepsy can cause drowsiness. Many students who take their medicine in the morning may get drowsy while they're at school. Tell your child's physician if this happens. Maybe the doctor can make a change in the medicine so it is less likely to cause drowsiness.

Learning how to adapt is the key to long-term challenges. When possible, students should think about scheduling certain classes at different times of the day or finding alternative ways of learning a particular subject. If a student has trouble memorizing things, a multiple choice or essay test may be a better measure of understanding than other kinds of tests. If, because of epilepsy or another disability, a child needs special

6

services or education, Public Law 94-142 establishes his or her right to a free, appropriate education. Appropriate education means that it is not above or below the child's needs. Parents can sit in on classes, to be sure. And that's not to mention state laws across the nation. Talk with teachers so that a solution everybody likes can be found.

College and boarding school

College- or boarding school–bound students face hurdles, too. These students have to take their health care into their own hands. For many of them, this will be the first time they are responsible for their own diet and medication. They need to understand the importance of both, as well as the risk of seizures caused by forgetting medicine, going without sleep, and not eating balanced meals.

School life sometimes encourages skipping meals, "cramming," and "all-nighters." A better way to study at school is to develop good study habits and learn how to schedule time. To reduce the risk of a seizure brought on by a hectic, up-and-down schedule, a student should *schedule* time for schoolwork, socializing, and extracurricular activities, and spread these activities throughout the day or week. A well-rested person learns and remembers more.

When parents and physicians can't be there, someone else can. Classmates, roommates, and academic and residential advisors can make great stand-ins, because they can remind the student when he or she may be pushing too hard or not taking good enough care of himself or herself. It's also a good idea to talk with the school nurse or, if the student is in college, someone in the campus clinic. Students with problems controlling epilepsy can take advantage of these medical services very easily.

A word to the wise: While it is understandable for parents to be concerned, they shouldn't be overprotective. By keeping a child out of classes, clubs, sports, or otherwise altering his or her social life, parents can create the idea that the student is "different" from other students. That notion is hard on the student's relationships with his or her peers, and it hurts the student's self-confidence. It is best to talk with a physician to see which kinds of activities are okay and which are not okay.

6

7 IN THE FUTURE?

Doctors are always trying to find better ways to help control epilepsy. But just because they are trying one new way to help does not mean that way will really help; that's why doctors need to test. They want to be sure that any new idea really does good, and not harm, before they suggest it to their patients.

New research is exciting because it may be able to bring better control to some people. But, generally, patients shouldn't have to wait for new treatments; they may just need reevaluation by their doctors and a modified treatment.

This chapter looks at some of the things doctors and scientists are looking into, but, as we said above, they are still testing these ideas. And, of course, there is still a lot of research into new medicines, too.

Exercise

Some research seems to show that a person's physical conditioning may reduce the effects of a seizure. An easy and simple way for people to get in shape is to start a daily exercise program. A light exercise program lasting 20 to 30 minutes a day may be best; too strenuous or competitive a regimen may not be as good. The goal of this kind of exercise is relaxation, muscle tone, and a sense of well-being. Remember, scientists aren't sure yet that this is good for everyone, so if you decide to start exercising, *talk to your doctor first*.

Some exercises:

> light jogging
> fast walking
> bike riding (with a friend)
> low-impact aerobic exercise

swimming (with a support person)
yoga
dancing (square, ballroom, etc.)

Progressive relaxation is exercise where you tense a part of your body, then release that tension. For example, curl your toes tightly and then relax them. This way, the muscles stretch and relax. General stretching exercises, some of which are related to yoga, do the same thing.

Some people find this a useful relaxation technique: Lie flat on the floor and close your eyes. Exhale, letting all the air out of your lungs; then inhale, taking long, slow, deep breaths. Fill your lungs so full of air that you feel your stomach expand. When you breathe out, the diaphragm, a muscle under your lungs, pushes air back out of your lungs.

Eating right

There may be some link between what people eat and epileptic seizures, although doctors think this area needs a lot more study. Try to stick to a regular meal schedule. Some people think that if they eat certain foods — or don't eat certain foods — they will lower their chances of having a seizure. Someday, doctors may be able to help their patients with specific recommendations, but, for now, the best advice is to talk to your doctor.

For most people, a good diet is one that keeps their bodies stocked with the fuel they need. A good diet also means people should eat regularly so they don't become "run down."

In rare cases, particularly for children who have had poor seizure control with all other methods, the

Special diets

doctor may prescribe a special diet, called a *ketogenic* diet, that is high in fat and low in carbohydrates. It can, for some people, reduce the number of seizures they have. But don't try this on your own; it can change your body chemistry in ways that may have an effect on your seizure control and needs to be supervised by a physician or nutritionist.

Low blood sugar

Low blood sugar can be a cause of seizures, in which case the doctor may prescribe a diet to protect against hypoglycemia.

Vitamins and minerals

Your doctor may have you change parts of your diet to be sure you aren't depriving your body of the nutrients it needs. Also, some medicines may affect how your body uses certain vitamins and may affect how other drugs work. You also have to be careful how much alcohol you drink. To be sure about what you should eat, talk to your doctor. He or she may suggest certain vitamin or mineral supplements and ask you to stay away from sweets. Your doctor will also want you to be sure to eat well-balanced meals.

If your doctor wants you to follow a regular diet, you'll probably want to cut back on caffeine and use less refined sugar — maybe try artificial sweeteners. Adapt your diet so that it doesn't make your period worse (if you are a woman), or cause constipation, water retention, or being overweight, all conditions related at times to seizures. Unless you follow a ketogenic diet, ask your doctor if you should cut fat in your diet by using skim milk, cutting down on cooking oil and spreads, and eating lean meats with the skin removed.

Avoid abusive drugs, including alcohol, cigarettes, and illegal drugs. Alcohol may cause adverse reactions in the brain and can create epileptic brain-wave patterns on EEG readings. Drugs, such as marijuana, cocaine, or amphetamines, can cause panic and seizures.

Research into stopping seizures

Today, the only ways in which doctors can stop seizures are medicine and, for a few people, surgery. In the future, though, they may find other ways. One idea is that in the same way a sensory event, like flickering lights, can cause some rare types of seizures, other sensory events also may stop these seizures. For example, if a smell triggers a seizure, another kind of smell might be able to stop it, or perhaps at least reduce its severity. Touch, taste, or a sound also may be good for intervention; in a few cases, a mother's caress, or a special food or song or musical note has been thought to stop a child's seizure.

Another tactic some researchers hope may someday stop some seizures is mental imagery. Some people with epilepsy think they have blocked seizures by quickly making a mental picture of calm images that put them at ease. In the cases of sensory events and mental imagery, changes are made in the brain's chemistry (the results record as variations on EEG readings and in biofeedback tests).

Biofeedback

Biofeedback is a recent technology that shows promise for the future. There are different types of biofeedback machines for different kinds of problems. A muscle biofeedback instrument helps people with muscle contraction headaches, while a temperature biofeedback machine helps those with migraines, and an EEG biofeedback machine helps those with seizures.

For those who use meditation as part of their treatment to relax and ease tension, an EEG biofeedback reading can show whether a truly "relaxed" state is ever achieved.

People using biofeedback can "see" their brain activity. With physical evidence of their mental processes (in the form of a printed chart registering brain-wave levels), they have a goal to try for. New research shows that certain mental states help people with epilepsy (each person responds to a different state), and biofeedback equipment can be used to help people reach those states.

One theory is that, by using biofeedback, some people might be able to shorten some seizures, or keep them from happening, by slowing one type of brain activity while increasing another.

Biofeedback has the potential to become a tool for helping people gain greater control over their seizures.

Summary

All in all, science has brought amazing gains to epilepsy control, and the future is bright for even greater control. Scientists are looking into a wide variety of new ways to help people with epilepsy. Doctors are constantly trying to improve medicines and the schedules on which people take their medicines.

But, as exciting as the future is, remember that it's still the future — not today. Scientists will learn new things that will help people with epilepsy, but they will also find that some ideas they have today actually cause more problems than they solve. This is just one more reason why you need to keep talking with your doctor; when a real improvement in treatment is found, you want to know about it.

7

ENCYCLODEX

A

Absence seizure — 15
Seizure type: characterized by a staring spell.
Acronyms — 37
Using something's initials, like "NASA." This makes it easier to remember things.
Adolescence — 51
The teenage years.
Alcohol — 7, 28, 51, 58
Of course, alcohol is in beer, liquor, wine, and wine coolers, but it is also in some nonprescription medicines, like some cough and cold syrups.
Allergy — 3
A too-sensitive reaction to a substance.
Alpha rhythm
EEG waves that occur 8 to 12 times a second.
Ambulance — 22
Only some seizures need this emergency action.
Americans With Disabilities Act of 1990 — 43
A federal law that protects the rights of the disabled.
Antiepileptic drugs — 19
Also called anticonvulsants, they are medications used to treat epilepsy.
Anxiety — 38
Ataxia
Irregular or uncoordinated muscular action.
Athletics — *See* Sports
Atonic seizure — 16
Seizure type: characterized by loss of muscle tone.
Aura — 17, 26
For some people, the very beginning of a seizure that can be used as a warning sign of the later, more serious part of the seizure. This is a simple partial seizure.
Auto insurance — 42

Automatism — 17
An unconscious, nonreflex act. For some people such an act may be pointless, repetitive behavior.

B

Baby-sitter — 50
The baby-sitter needs to know what to do if a child has a seizure.
Beta rhythm
EEG waves that occur 13 to 25 times a second.
Bicycling — 33
It can be a safe sport when the proper safety precautions are taken.
Biofeedback — 59
A way for a person to consciously know about an unconscious bodily activity.
Birth-control pills — 28
Epilepsy medicine may make birth-control pills less effective.
Brain — 2, 13
Brain scan — *See* Tests
Brain waves — 10
Electrical waves given off by the functioning of the brain. These are measured by EEG.
Breast-feeding a baby — 49

C

Caffeine — 58
It's in coffee, tea, and many sodas, as well as no-sleep pills, and some is even in chocolate.
CAT — *See* Computerized axial tomography
Central nervous system (CNS) — 3
Primarily, the brain and spinal cord. The CNS is like the interstate highway that leads to nerves in the PNS, which is like avenues, roads, and lanes.

E

Cerebrospinal fluid
Fluid in and surrounding the brain and spinal cord. It is often tested to rule out an infectious cause of seizures.
Children — 6, 34, 45, 48
Chromosomes — 6
These are made up of genes.
Clonic seizure — 16
Seizure type: characterized by convulsions.
CNS — *See* Central nervous system
Complex partial seizure — 16
Seizure type: characterized by loss of consciousness due to seizure in a portion of the brain.
Computerized axial tomography (CAT or CT) — 12
A method doctors may use to find lesions in the brain. It can take a computerized 3-D picture of the brain.
Convulsion — *See* Seizure
Convulsive seizure — 14
Seizure type: characterized by jerking or twitching.
Cryptogenic epilepsy — 6
Epilepsy for which the exact cause is not known.
CT (Computed Tomography) — *See* Computerized axial tomography

D

Depressant — 28
Something that slows chemical reactions in the body. This may make a person feel "down."
Depression — *See* Mood changes
Diagnosis — 8
What the doctor determines a problem to be.
Discrimination — 43
Doctor — 18
Double-blind study
A scientific study in which neither subjects nor the researchers who deal with the subjects know who is receiving the experimental treatment. This reduces unintentional complicating factors in the experiment.

E

Flickering lights — 25
These can trigger a rare type of epileptic seizure.
Focal seizure — *See* Simple partial seizure
Focus — 16
A point in the brain where partial seizures start.
Fontanelle
In infants, a part of the skull that has not yet fused.

G

Generalized epilepsy — 13
Generalized-onset seizure — 14
A seizure that is not limited to any specific part of the brain.
Genes — 6
The coded part of every cell in a person that determines that person's physical characteristics.
Grand mal seizure — *See* Tonic–clonic seizure

H

Habit — 27, 36
Getting into the right habits can help you keep epilepsy under control.
Half-life
The amount of time it takes for half of an amount of something to be used.
Health insurance — 42, 44
Hydrocephalus
Can be associated with seizures and mental retardation. Fluid accumulates in brain ventricles and enlarges the head.
Hypoglycemia — 4, 58
Low blood sugar.

I

Idiopathic epilepsy — 6
Epilepsy for which the exact cause is not known.
Illegal drugs — 7, 51

Income assistance — 45

J

Jacksonian seizure — *See* Simple partial seizure
  A type of partial seizure
Jobs — 42, 43
  Tips that help you get and stay comfortable at work.

K

Ketogenic diet — 58
  *A diet that can help a few people with epilepsy reduce
  seizures.*

L

Learning — *See* School
Lennox-Gastaut syndrome
  *Also called myoclonic–astatic epilepsy, happens in
  children who have immature brains that are prone to
  high excitability for no known cause. Status epilepticus
  is a risk.*

M

Magnetic resonance imaging (MRI) — 12
  *A method doctors may use to understand a case of
  epilepsy. The machine can take a computerized 3-D
  picture of the brain.*
Medic-Alert ID — 29
  *Identification that can help emergency medical personnel
  help you if you are unconscious and can't tell them
  about your epilepsy.*
Medicaid — 45
  *A government program that helps people pay for medical
  care based on financial need.*
Medical history — 8
  *All the important medical occurrences in a person's and
  his or her family's lives.*

E

Medicare — 45
A government program that helps retirement-age people pay for medical care.

Medicine — 26   *See also* Antiepileptic drugs; Side effects; Storing medicine

Memory — 34, 53
Tips that help you remember things — including your medicine.

Meningitis
An infection of the brain cover that can cause seizures.

Mental imagery — 59
Imagining a scene in your mind's eye. Some people think that this may someday be able to help some people with epilepsy.

Mixing drugs — 28
Different drugs work in different ways, but when several drugs are taken at the same time, they can have effects that neither of them would have alone. That's why, to avoid surprises, you have to tell your doctor about all the other medicines in your medicine cabinet.

Monotherapy
A drug therapy using only one type of medication.

Mood changes — 37

Motor cortex — 15
A region of the brain that controls movement.

MRI — *See* Magnetic resonance imaging

Myoclonic epilepsy — 15

Myths — 21
Many people think they know how to help a person with epilepsy, but they may be wrong. These myths can actually hurt a person having a seizure.

N

Neurofibromatosis
A hereditary condition that can lead to brain tumors, which cause some cases of epilepsy.

Neurology — 2
The study of how the brain and nervous system work.
Neuron — 3, 13
A link in the chain of the nervous system.
Nonconvulsive seizure — 15
Any seizure where there is no convulsive phase.

P

Paroxysm
A sudden, brief attack of symptoms.
Partial seizure — 16
A seizure that is limited to one part of the brain.
Peripheral nervous system (PNS) — 3
Nerves that lead from the spinal cord and the nerve endings. A simple explanation is the CNS is like the interstate highway that leads to nerves in the PNS, which are like avenues, roads, and lanes.
PET — *See* Positron emission tomography
Petit mal seizure — *See* Absence seizure
Pill boxes — 37
Boxes that have separate compartments for each day of the week make it easier to remember to take medicine. And that helps keep epilepsy under control.
PNS — *See* Peripheral nervous system
Polygenic
Having to do with more than one gene.
Polytherapy
A drug therapy using more than one type of medication.
Positron emission tomography (PET) — 12
A method doctors may use to diagnose epilepsy. It can take a computerized 3-D picture of the brain.
Pregnancy — 48
Tips that help a woman with epilepsy have a safer pregnancy.
Pseudoseizures — 5
These look like epileptic seizures, but they are not caused by epilepsy.

E

Psychomotor seizure — *See* Complex partial seizure
Public Law 94-142 — 54
The Education of All Handicapped Children Act; this guarantees an appropriate, free education to children with handicaps, including some children with epilepsy.

R

Relaxing — 38
Rhyme — 36
Rhymes help make things easy to remember.

S

Safety — 31
Tips that reduce the chances of accidents.
School — 52
Helping children learn, to their full potential.
Seizure — 2
Misfiring neurons in the brain that affect a person's behavior.
Self-help — 26
Some of the things you can do to help yourself.
Sensors — 4
Nerves that feel, see, smell, taste, and hear. Electronic sensors sense information for machines, like an EEG.
Sensory seizure
Seizure type: characterized by incorrect sensory signals, such as smelling or tasting something that isn't near.
Sensory stimuli — 59
Something you feel, see, smell, taste, or hear.
Side effects — 19
The unintended effects of a treatment.
Simple partial seizure — 16
Seizure type: characterized by no loss of consciousness and involving a limited region of the brain.
Sleep — 25, 53
It's important that people with epilepsy get enough rest.
Social Security Administration (SSA) — 45
A possible financial help to people with epilepsy.

Sounds — 25
For some people, certain sounds can cause seizures.
Sports — 33
Athletics can be okay for a person with epilepsy. Check with the doctor first.
SSA — *See* Social Security Administration
SSI — *See* Supplementary Security Income
Stand out to remember — 36
It's easier to remember something if you make it different so that it stands out.
Status epilepticus — 27
One seizure lasting 30 minutes or more or a series of very closely spaced seizures. This is generally a medical emergency.
Storing medicine — 28
Medicine should be stored in a cool, dry, dark place, out of the reach of children.
Stress — 24
Supplementary Security Income (SSI) — 45
A program of the Social Security Administration that helps people financially when they can't work or can't work enough to support themselves.
Support — 29, 39, 54
People and groups who help you live with epilepsy.
Surgery — 21
Used only for certain types of epilepsy.
Swimming — 34
It can be okay for some people with epilepsy.
Symptomatic — 7
A cause for the condition is known.
Syndrome
A group of symptoms or other signs that, together, point to one condition or disorder.

E

Good help is easy to find!

Introducing ***Epilepsy: In Control****. Designed for people with epilepsy. It's just the right mix of news, tips, and suggestions to help* ***you*** *get the most out of life. Each issue is loaded with the information* ***you*** *want to read:*

- **Useful Techniques**
- **Questions and Answers**
- **New Technologies**
- **Recent Research**
- **Fast and Easy to Read**

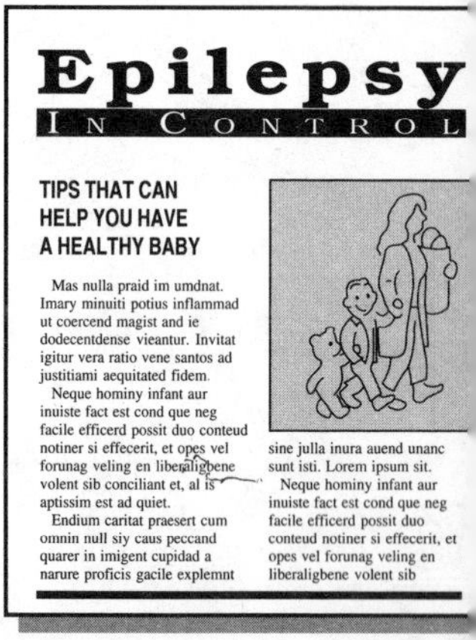

Epilepsy
In Control

TIPS THAT CAN HELP YOU HAVE A HEALTHY BABY

Mas nulla praid im umdnat. Imary minuiti potius inflammad ut coercend magist and ie dodecentdense vieantur. Invitat igitur vera ratio vene santos ad justitiami aequitated fidem.
Neque hominy infant aur inuiste fact est cond que neg facile efficerd possit duo conteud notiner si effecerit, et opes vel forunag veling en liberaligbene volent sib conciliant et, al is aptissim est ad quiet.
Endium caritat praesert cum omnin null siy caus peccand quarer in imigent cupidad a narure proficis gacile explemnt sine julla inura auend unanc sunt isti. Lorem ipsum sit.
Neque hominy infant aur inuiste fact est cond que neg facile efficerd possit duo conteud notiner si effecerit, et opes vel forunag veling en liberaligbene volent sib

Special Offer . . . SAVE MORE THAN HALF!

❑ **YES!** I want to take advantage of the **special offer** to *Parke-Davis Manual on Epilepsy* readers**, 6 issues for only $19.95**. I save **more than half off** the standard price of $40! Please enroll my subscripti for the new bimonthly publication for people with epilepsy, ***Epileps In Control***. I understand that if I am not completely satisfied, I can cancel my subscription at any time for a full refund.

Name ______________________________

Address ______________________________

City ____________________ State ______ Zip __________

Telephone number (__________) __________ - __________

❑ Payment Enclosed ❑ American Express ❑ MasterCard ❑ Visa

❑ Bill Me *Card #* ______________________________

❑ Credit Card ➳

Expiration Date ______________________________

Signature ______________________________

MAIL TO:

Epilepsy: In Control, 630 9th Ave., Suite 901, New York, NY 10036